HOW TO LOOK YOUNGER

- Get a Younger Skin Naturally –

Feeling Beautiful in Your Own Skin

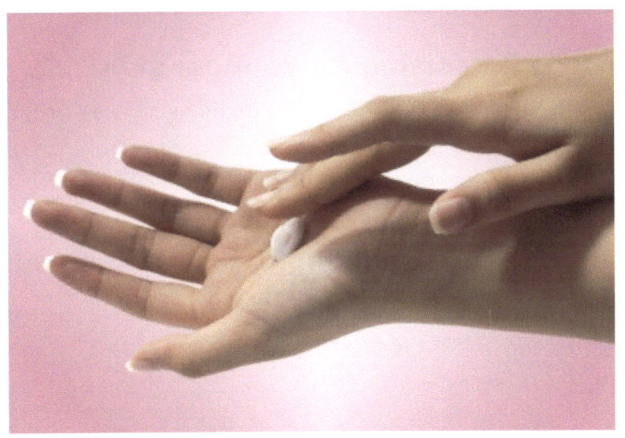

P. Karn

Table of Contents

Introduction

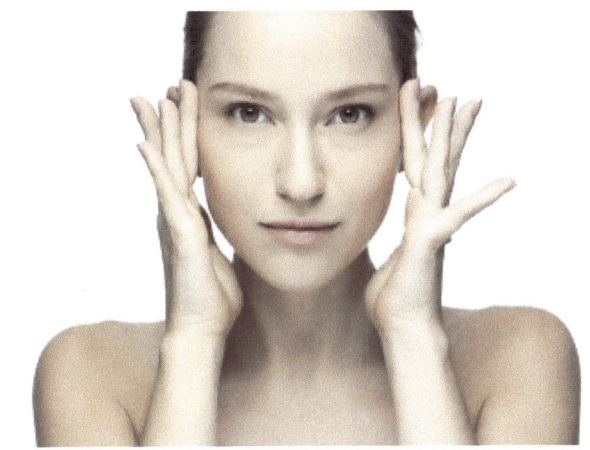

As human beings, it is natural to want and look for quick fixes, an easy way out even when it is our health we put at risk. But are they the best option really?

Do you feel uncomfortable in your own skin?

We all have that friend whose skin never seems to age or blemish in whatever condition. Worse still, they do not have to try hard to keep their skin looking fresh and younger. On the other hand, you have tried to move heaven and earth to bring your skin condition to match that of your friend but to no avail. Oh, believe me I have been there and I understand how this feels.

Even with the most amazing body, the lack of beautiful skin can often make you feel incomplete. I have found that in life there is nothing as sad as not being able to feel comfortable in your own skin.

With these economically unfriendly ages, it is no longer as easy as it used to be to have a dermatologist of skin specialist on speed dial. I have also discovered that DIY sounds better that IOU, and I bet you agree too. Indeed hard economic times call for more affordable measures.

Where is the need of spending hundreds of dollars or even thousands for a better skin tone when you can do it absolutely free?

So, you have tried everything from cosmetic surgery to chemical based formulas but nothing seems to work for your skin. It is not because you are doing it the wrong way but it is because you are using all the wrong products.

I have discovered that regardless of all the anti-aging promises we are offered by consumer products, nothing quite beats natural skin care products. There are so many benefits you can reap from using natural products; especially in this cancer prone era.

The last thing you want is to bring skin cancer upon yourself. This is exactly what most, if not all of these chemical based skin products and procedures will bring upon you. If you are lucky enough, you may escape with just a few side effects that will take you some time to correct.

If you are like me and fear for your dear life and skin, this e-book is for you. With the insights I share with you, you will be able to see that the answer to amazing skin was right under your nose or maybe in your home this entire time.

Come with me on this great journey and discover natural ways to always keep your skin young and gorgeous.

Chapter 1: My motivation

The Secret behind My Naturally Beautiful Skin

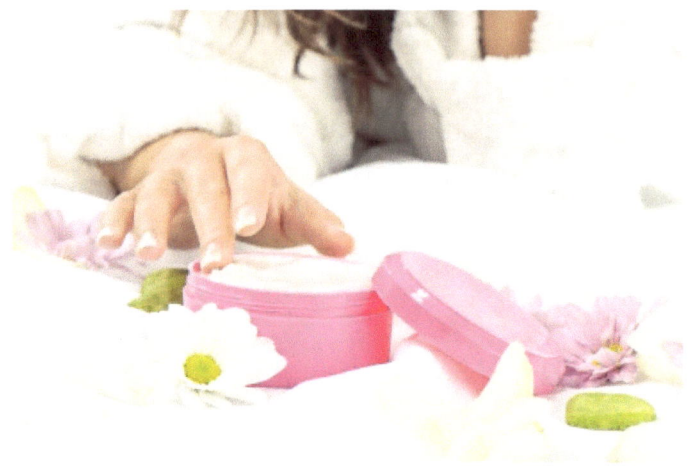

It is every woman's dream to have naturally flawless, shinny skin but very few actually have such skin types.

I happen to fall under the not so lucky bunch that has to make the skin thing happen for them through other means.

At a young age I became very conscious about my not so appealing skin type. Throughout school, especially high school I was more of a weirdo than a cool kid. I would wear clothes that covered most of my skin and I would flood my face with make up to cover the 'imperfections' as I saw them.

In college I discovered I could enjoy wearing clothes that showed a bit of skin but I would have to cover my 'flaws' using skin masks. This was rather expensive for my pockets but I wanted to live like any other woman. If this was the cost then I was more than happy to oblige!

After college I got a job that paid well and this opened up a whole world of opportunities.

Now, I could afford most procedures and products that promise amazing skin results. I must say life was good, at least I thought so. What I did not know was that with all these procedures, there comes a time when your skin will simply stop to respond and this is disastrous for any woman. Lucky for me, I got out before it was too late and you can too.

You can ask your skin specialist but I bet that they will not tell you this, least they risk losing you and your money.

As a woman, I have found that one of the most important aspects of my beauty is my skin. I have done it all; from Botox to using chemical based skin creams. All this was for one common goal, to avoid the wrinkles and look younger for longer. I would only be lying if I told you that all these means and ways do not work, because they do, but only for so long.

Over time, I got tired of the frequent visits to the doctor and the countless injection you get on your face and other body parts all in the effort to look younger. Plus I realized that the people, who have gone under the knife or under the syringe for the purposed or remaining young end up looking well, deformed. Not in an abnormal way but in some way, I'm sure you understand.

I had always read about natural ways of keeping the skin healthy and looking younger. However, I always brushed them off and thought to myself, why should I go to all the trouble when there is an easy way out? And the easy way I took.

With this observation and knowledge the last thing I wanted was to look like most people I know or some stars on TV. And so, I decided to start on a journey and try out different natural ways to keep my skin healthy and natural. I admit it was hard at first but I made it through and this is how I was able to write this e-book.

You, my dear reader are lucky because you do not have to struggle like I did in the beginning. I was able to separate the good and the bad to offer you the best ways to enjoy beautifully natural skin using acts you can incorporate easily in your day to day life.

If you have been struggling with skin issues and like me you have tried all means and ways to no avail, this e-book is for you!

By following the doctrines I teach you, not only will you be able to have younger looking skin, but you will be able to do it the healthy way.

The Teachings to Naturally Beautiful Skin

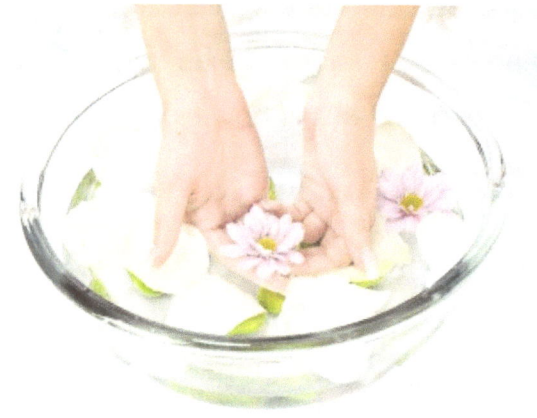

Just like any other aspect of life, you need to be dedicated to something for it to work for you. You have probably tried natural skin care products but you never use them long enough to find out whether they work. Take it from me, they do work. Actually, they work better than all skin care creams and procedures I have ever used.

In order to enjoy naturally beautiful skin, it will take so much more than applying homemade masks. It goes deeper to:

- Adapting healthy eating habits.

- Striving to remain physically fit.

- Taking time to care for your skin.

These are the three areas we are going to cover in this e-book.

Let's get going, shall we…..

Chapter 2: Your Diet and Your Skin

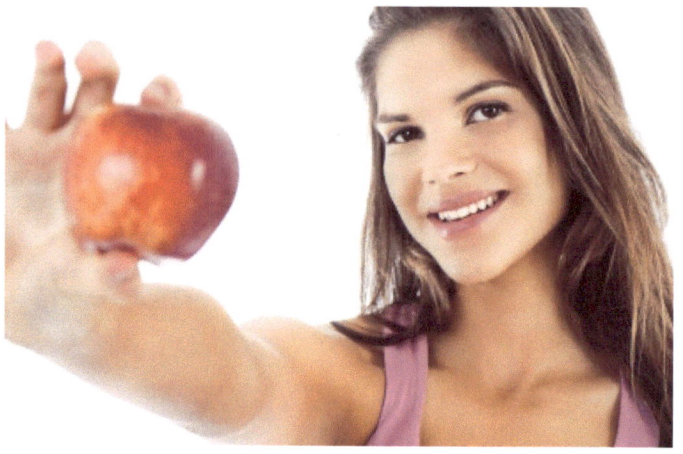

Overall, to be able to have a naturally healthy and younger skin, you need to adopt good habits when it comes to nutrition. Most of us eat four to five meals every day. If you ensure that all these meals are healthy, you will have made the first step towards ensuring your skin stays naturally younger.

Healthy Eating and how it is Relevant to Your Skin

As the saying goes, you are what you eat!

The thing about our skins is that even if you were born with the most beautiful healthy skin, if you adopt bad eating habits you will damage your skin.

Our diet is a very significant aspect in our skin care. I can go on and on about ways to take care for your skin. However, it will make no difference if I do not teach you how to care for it through your diet.

Actually, in my journey to naturally younger skin, I found that diet was the most important aspect. I realized that even if I got the other parts rights, without a good dietary guideline is was all in vain. Plus, this is probably the easiest part because we all love eating, or maybe I'm just speaking for myself. Either way, you need a proper dietary plan if you want your skin to age gracefully.

It is very important for us to eat foods that cater for our well being and this includes the skin. A good meal that is beneficial to your skin should be balanced. Strive to balance vitamins, minerals, fats, carbohydrates as well as proteins. Ensure you have leafy greens in all your meals. You should include fruits and sprouts in your daily diet.

When you include the right amounts of foods in your meals, it not only becomes easy for you to enjoy silky and younger skin but also maintain great overall health. You are able to avoid skin pimples, acne and other blemishes.

The dietary dos and don'ts of for younger skin

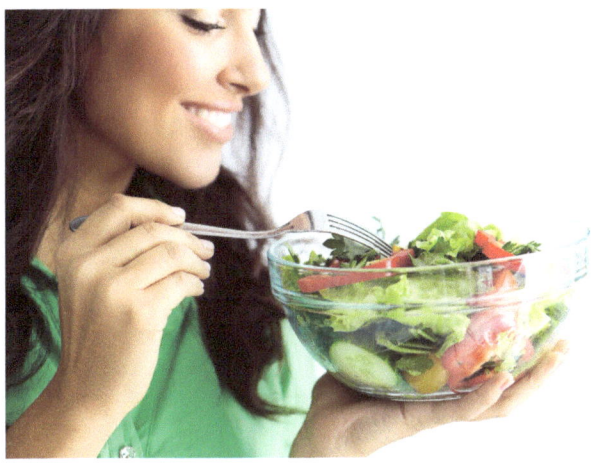

Have you ever met someone for the first time and you get chatting. Somewhere in the middle of the conversation you are made to state your age; albeit willingly. The minute you utter it, you realize that the other person's jaw is almost dropping. They are surprised and by impulse they say, I actually thought you were older. They try to sugar coat the 'you look older than you are' but the damage is already done.

It is not their fault because they said it as it is. I'm going to tell you this for free, part of the reason you look older is because you are not taking enough care for your skin. You will probably eat anything that you set your taste buds on without second thought. I know this how? I have been there too. Actually part of my wake-up call was the fact that people thought I was older than I actually looked. Despite my ridiculously hot body, can you imagine? I bet you can. Hahaaa!

In order to enjoy healthier skin that makes you look younger than you are, there are things you need to incorporate in your meals while others you need to steer clear of.

The dos for a younger skin

Ensure that all your meals contain carbohydrates, proteins and vitamins. These are the three food types that are known to aid in skin care. If you find that your skin is saggy and looks aged than your actual age, you need to increase the amounts of these foods in your diet.

Proteins – for a youthful glow

You can get proteins from a number of foods. White meat and red meat are the known sources of proteins. For vegetarians, proteins can be found in legumes like beans, sprouts and dairy products. Soya products are also very ideal and are rich sources of protein. Soya is readily available in different forms like granules, soya chunks and flour. They are very healthy for the skin.

Vitamins – for a smooth texture

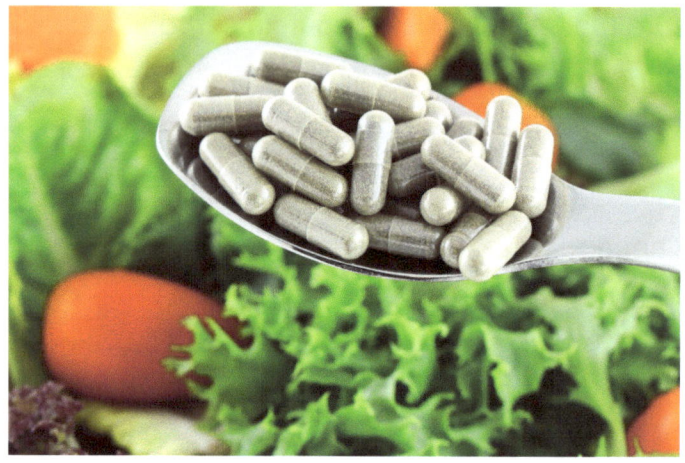

Vitamins play an important role in skin care. The most important vitamin types are vitamin A, C, B, D and vitamin E. these vitamins come from different sources and they ought to be included in your daily meals.

Sources of Vitamin A include - mangoes, radish, and apples. This vitamin helps to reconstruct the tissues of the skin and it also detoxifies the skin. When the skin is detoxified, it is protected from pimples, acne and other blemishes. This keeps it younger and clean.

Source of vitamin B include –you can get this vitamin from foods like vegetables; especially the green and leafy ones. This vitamin will boost your immune system and this keeps skin based conditions at bay. It is readily available in complex supplements like capsules that can be incorporated in your daily diet. This vitamin will also ensure you gain a fresh complexion.

Vitamin c sources – this is a very important vitamin. It fights and prevents allergies. It is very useful for the skin. Vitamin c nourishes the skin and keeps it radiant and younger. This vitamin will prevent further damage to the skin helping it to reconstruct and remain younger. With this vitamin I have been able to notice changes in my face as the wrinkles that had started being visible are slowly disappearing. You can get this vitamin from lemons, oranges, grapes and limes. You should include a glass of orange juice in your diet.

Sources of vitamin D – you can get this vitamin from dairy products and other sources of calcium. The main source of this vitamin is the sun, however, you need to bask before the sun gets too hot. The early morning sun is the best. This vitamin prevents break-out of skin conditions and it also nourishes the bones.

Vitamin E Sources – this vitamin smoothens and nourishes the skin keeping it young and lustrous. It also acts as sun screen. The sources of this vitamin include olives, butter, milk, dry fruits and fish. This vitamin prevents the drying of the skin. It also prevents the skin from getting patchy and saggy. You can also get this vitamin in form of capsules.

Carbohydrates – for clearer skin

When we hear carbohydrates, we assume that sugars are ideal for your skin but they are not. While sugar is a source of carbohydrates, it is not ideal for your skin as it causes more harm than good. The best source of carbohydrates is honey, jiggery or fruit sugar. Breads are also good sources of carbohydrates but you need to avoid white bread and instead go for brown bread as well as brown rice.

Most people do not get the right amounts of carbohydrates, proteins or vitamins and this leads to dull and saggy skin. It also leads to the pre-mature aging of the skin and you end up looking older than you are.

Water – keeps the skin hydrated

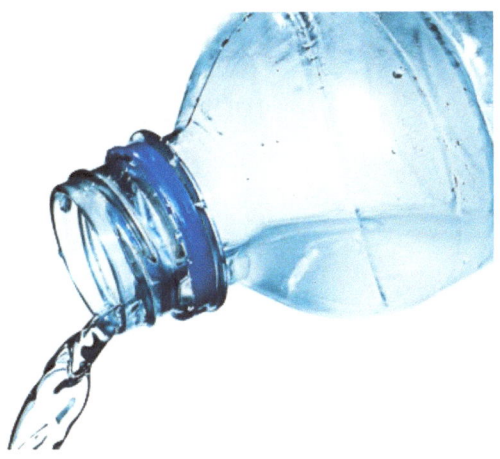

Skin cells are mostly made of water. When these cells lack adequate water the skin is dehydrated and looks perched and to some extent may even crack. Different people have different body water needs and thus I really would not force eight glasses of water down your throat.

For instance, I require four glasses of water daily. This is because most of the foods I eat are water based and this compensates my other four glasses. To be able to know how much water you require, just look at the foods you eat and try determine how much water is in there. Then compensate for the remaining glasses with pure water.

The point is that; ensure you take enough water to keep your skin hydrated. At least aim for eight glasses daily.

The don'ts for younger skin

If your plan to have a younger skin is going to come true, it will be partly because you avoided some dietary habits that are hazardous to your skin.

Some of the habits you need to steer clear of include:

- Taking in too much food than you actually need. In other words over-eating.

- Taking over processed meals that do not have any advantage to the body these include sugars.

- Taking junk foods like sweet pastries and fried foods.

The above habits lead to intestinal and body toxicity. When toxins are left to enter our bodies, they lead to skin damages and your skin wrinkles pre-maturely.

A sample eating plan for great skin

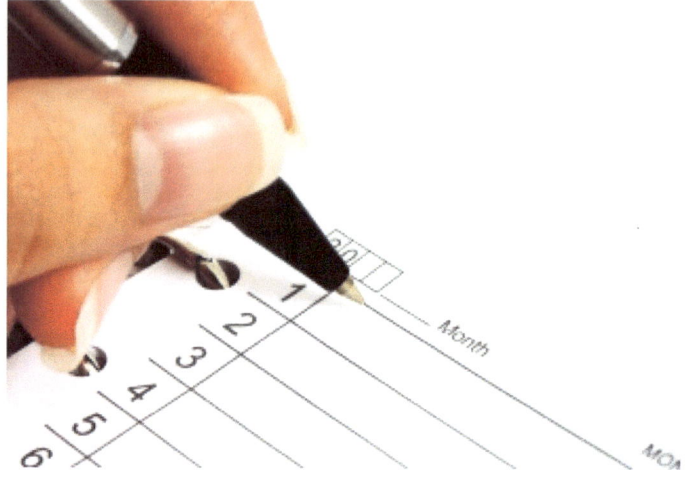

For breakfast

- A cup of fortified, whole grain cereal.

- A cup of skimmed milk.

- A cup of slices strawberries or grapefruits.

- A cup of green tea.

For lunch

- One serving of grilled chicken sandwich. Preferably made from chicken breast, tomatoes, whole grain bread, lettuce, a small portion of avocado and a teaspoon of mustard.

- An apple

- Water.

For dinner

- Wild salmon (5 oz)

- Spinach salad made from 2 cups of fresh spinach, half a cup of sliced red-bell pepper, half a cup of chopped tomato, half a cup of broccoli tossed with one tablespoon of balsamic vinegar and olive oil.

- Boiled potato.

- Water.

- A potion of any food that is a source of protein.

- Small bowl of Fruit salad.

It is clear to see that healthy eating is essential to a healthy, younger and glowing skin. By adhering to the dietary needs of your skin, you are able to look younger for longer. After a while you will notice that skin blemishes will start to disappear.

Believe, me, there is no better feeling than looking younger than you actually are. For the married ladies, your husband will fall in love with you all over again.

For the single ladies, don't be surprised if a younger guy hits on you.

With that said, our next chapter focuses on the exercises that help the skin to stay younger for longer.

Please turn over.....

Chapter 3: Exercising for younger skin

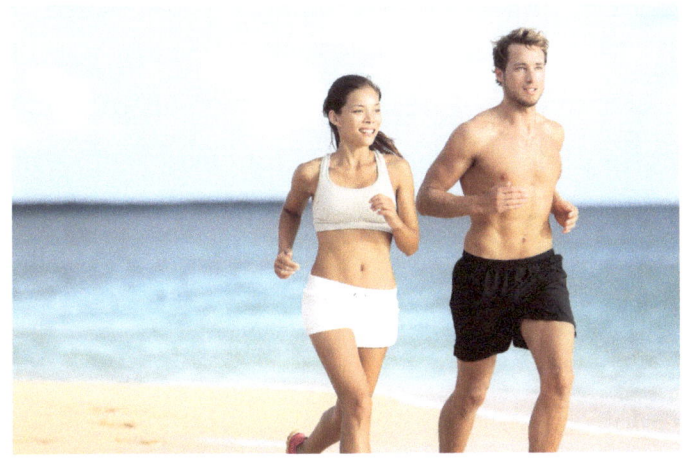

Just like any other health plan and I do not mean the insurance kind, exercising and your diet go hand in hand when it comes to caring for your skin. Regular exercising is one of the keys to healthy and younger skin.

You are probably reading this and you are like, I exercise often but it does not do anything for my skin. This is because you probably focus more on cardiovascular and weight management exercises and you forget to incorporate important anti-aging exercises like yoga and rest, yes rest is also an exercise when it comes to your skin.

So, how does exercise lead to healthy and younger skin?

I am going to tell you this for free, you cannot expect your skin to look its best if you do not incorporate exercise to your dietary plan. From exercising, I have been able to enjoy numerous benefits and I would like to share them with you.

The skin advantages from exercising

Circulation improvement

The reason you exercise is because it boosts blood circulation thereby helping the circulatory system and heart. What you did not know is that your skin requires a level of circulation to remain healthy and young too. What happens is, during exercise, the skin is nourished with blood flow and oxygen and this helps in reconstruction of the skin cells for better skin. The good thing is that this benefit is long term meaning your skin does not age quickly as the cells are regrouped often.

Reduction of stress

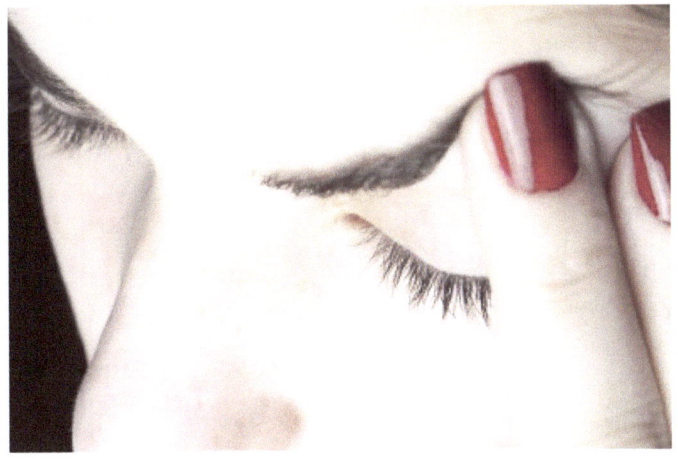

When you exercise, you reduce anxiety and stress. If you doubt the effect of stress on your skin, I ask you to observe the changes that take place on your skin when you are stressed. Personally, I develop pimples on my face and my skin dries up no matter how much water I take or how much fruits I eat. When I took up exercising, it was for weight management purposes. However, a friend of mine told me of the benefits it has to the skin and it motivated me to be working out even more. Stress causes intrinsic skin aging which appears sooner than it should. The best exercise for stress management is yoga, meditation and breathing exercise.

My all time favorite is the meditation and breathing exercise. Every time I meditate, I find that I come out of it less stressed and relaxed. To take this exercise:

- Sit upright with your legs crossed.

- Relax and free your mind of all thoughts.

- Breathe in and out deeply. Taking turn to block each nostril. Breathe in through one nostril while closing the other one with your fingers. Block the nostril you breathed through and breathe out using the other nostril.

- Alternate for five minutes and stop.

- Breathe in through both nostrils and exhale in the same way for a few minutes.

This completes the breathing part and now we enter the meditation part.

- Relax your body and muscles and free your mind.

I know I'm relaxed when I can hear my own heartbeat. You should too as a sign of relaxation.

- Think of happy thoughts. Try to think of something that brings you pleasure. It could be your child, family member, your job or even your home. Anything that makes you happy.

- Linger with that thought. This is called your mantra and you should be thinking of it each time you are meditating.

- Remain in the meditating state for at least half an hour every day.

When you get used to the meditation and breathing exercise, with time you will feel relived and it becomes hard to get stressed, which is a good thing for your skin. Actually, I always get out and perform my meditation and breathing whenever I feel as though in getting stressed over anything.

Getting adequate sleep

When you exercise, you actually activate your body and this ensures you sleep well at night as the body requires rest. This is because, during exercise, your body produces endorphins. These are hormones that help your body to enter into a mode of complete sleep at night. When you get adequate sleep, you body relaxes and your stress levels reduce. When you do fail to get enough sleep, your skin will also be unhealthy and it wrinkles faster than it should.

These are the skin benefits you get from exercising. So if you thought that your skin does not need exercises think again. Exercising helps your skin look great regardless of your age. Exercising also helps to boost longevity, physically, mentally and emotionally which are all important for your skin.

Clearly, the advantages of exercising are boundless. What are you waiting for? Let's get moving!

By now, you have a clear understanding of how essential it is for you to eat healthy diets and exercise for your skin. Indeed, these are the two factors that I find most helpful.

In our fourth and last chapter of this e-book, I will teach you of a good number of natural skin cleansers that go a long way in ensuring your skin remains younger for longer.

Turn over for natural skin treatments I bet you did not know.

The best part, you can make them at home using products you already have.

Chapter 4: Skin care using natural homemade treatments

How can I care for my skin without using chemical based treatments?

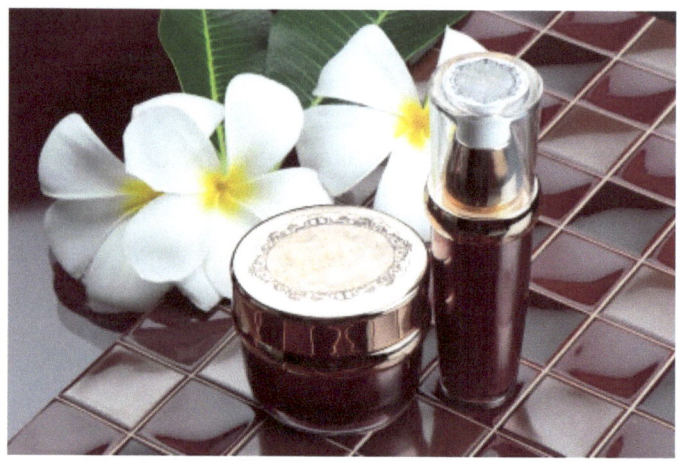

I can bet that this is the question lingering on your mind right now. Before I was able to determine what treatment options there are, all I could think of were the conventional aloe Vera treatment and use of natural soap. However, much to my disbelief, there are hundreds of skin treatment options that can be created from home using natural products.

I have been using these products and I must warn you, THEY ARE EXCEPTIONAL! I have never been happier and I have never looked younger. I am hooked for life and I love it.

Homemade facial cleansers

If you want to enjoy beautiful skin, especially facial skin, it is important for you to develop a habit of cleansing it at least twice every day. Personally, I wash my face in the morning and evening before bed.

You can make your very own natural facial cleanser. One does not have to spend a fortune for facial cleansers. Actually these chemical based cleansers are not ideal as they have several side effects on the skin.

Making of these natural skin cleansers require ingredients you already have at home. The first step towards creating cleansers is to know your skin type. Your face can be dry, oily or somewhere in between.

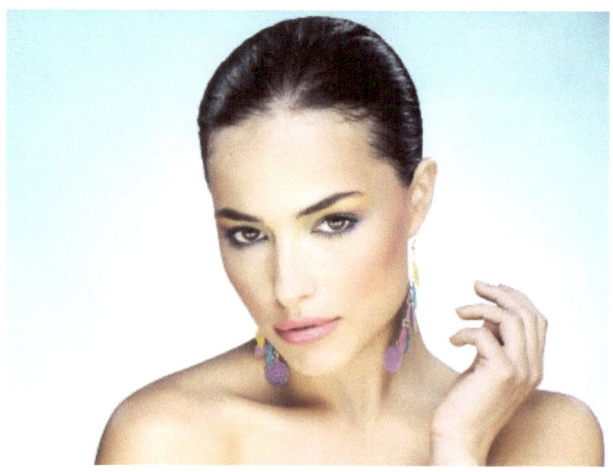

Natural Facial cleanser for oily skin

Since I have a dry skin, I had a friend of mine who tried out these facial cleansers for oily skin before I could actually write about them. They worked well for her. They can work for you too.

Oily skins are most prone to acne and thus require a facial cleanser that peels away the dead dry skin. There are numerous home ingredients that contain alphahydroxy acids which are ideal for exfoliating the skin. These include apple juice, milk, vinegar, pineapples, oranges, lemon juice, grapes and even tomatoes.

To make a facial cleanser from these products, you need to mix one type with either baking soda or egg white. Make a pasty blend and apply on the skin. Wash off after a few minutes. This will strip off dirt and open up the pores for a smooth silky skin. When you develop a habit off cleansing your face with homemade products, you will enjoy youthful skin always.

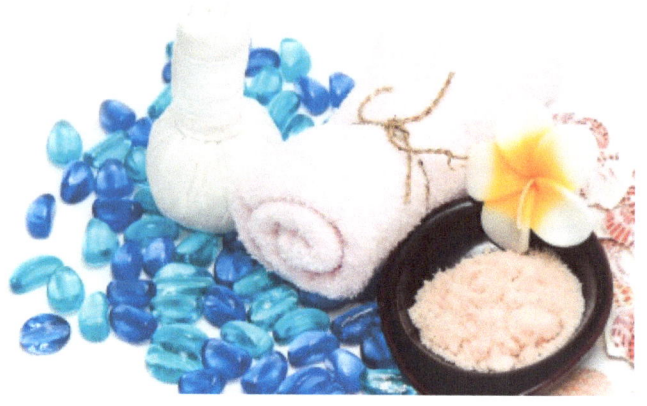

Natural Facial cleanser for dry skin

I have a dry skin and so these natural homemade cleansers come in handy. If you saw my face, you would not know it is the dry type.

If you share my sentiments, you need cleansers that heal, soothe and moisturize your skin. Such products are like aloe Vera, honey, cream, milk as well as green tea. These offer great skin cleansing possibilities.

My all time favorite cleanser is the mixture of milk/yogurt and honey. The reason as to why I like it so much is because I can eat a bit of it before I apply it on my body. These blends can be used for years and years. I have personally used it for close to five years now and it never fails to impress.

Before applying the mixture, dip it (of course in a bowl or bottle) in hot water until it is warm enough. This allows the honey to mix well with the milk or yogurt. Shake it and apply.

Green tea can be mixed with yogurt and applied on the skin. Green tea is an anti-oxidant and anti-inflammatory and is very gentle on the skin.

Actually, I have used it severally and I find it very therapeutic. The feeling I get afterwards is simply relaxing.

Natural Cleansers for normal skin

These cleansers are not only ideal for normal skin but also the two skin types we have mentioned above. This cleanser is made from oatmeal mixed with water, milk or yogurt. Oatmeal makes your skin glow and it is an exfoliating product.

Grind some oatmeal using your blender and mix it with water that is a third of your oat mixture. This will help to create a paste. Apply on your skin and allow it to dry. Rinse off using warm water.

Did you know that ground coffee is an exceptional treatment for any skin type? Now you do. The next time you make your coffee do not toss out the coffee grounds ad these are amazing whole body scrub.

These coffee remains will scrub off dead skin cells to leave your skin all fine and smooth.

I realized this as I was making my morning coffee one day and the texture of the coffee grounds felt nice on the hands, so I tried it on my face for a few days. I must admit, I was a tad bit scared but the result was amazing. So with time I tried it on my entire body and I loved it, still do.

Apart from leaving the skin in finesse, it also tightens the pores and this leads to smooth skin. You can add olive oil (extra virgin) if you have dry skin. This can be your weekly treat.

Helpful tip – since getting yogurt to apply to the whole body can be expensive, you can use water in place of milk and yogurt. Once you have created a paste add a bit of yogurt or milk and honey. This ensures you get a cleanser with all the nutrients for a cheaper cost. However, your skin deserves a treat every now and then. Personally, I budget for the yogurt or milk and honey treatment every two weeks. The rest of the time I use the water based cleanser.

Plus, each time you rinse off the cleansers, always use warm water. This is because warm water has a soothing effect on the skin.

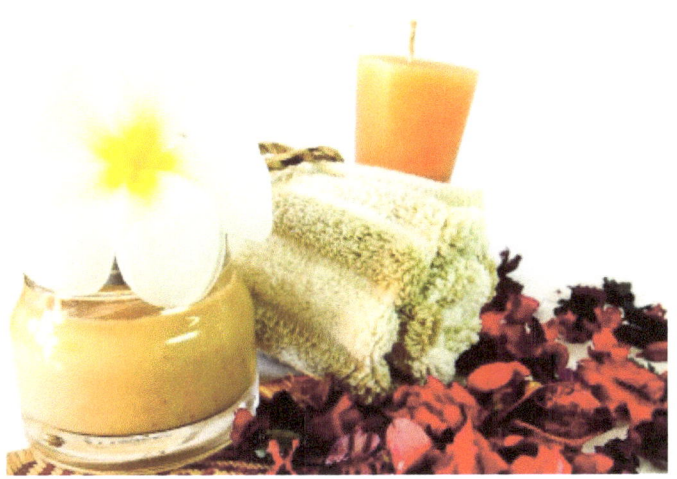

Using oil based cleansers

Let me clear up a misconception you among many people may have. Oil does NOT cause skin acne. There are numerous factors that contribute to development of acne like adolescent age, clogged pores and hormones. Actually a good combination of oil can clean, protect and moisturize your skin; regardless of the type.

The best oil types for facial cleansing are olive oil (especially the extra virgin type) and castor oil. You can mix the two for amazing results. The castor oil will clean while the olive oil moisturizes. Alternatives can be grape seed oil, jojoba oil and tea tree oil for people with acne.

Apply the mixture using the palm of your hand and leave it for a while. Use warm water and a cloth to sponge your skin. This opens the pores and allows the oil mixture to penetrate and work its magic. Relax for a while and use warm water to rinse off the oil mixture.

Other amazing sources of natural skin cleansers include papaya, crushed strawberries, rose oil, sea salt, juniper berry oil, marigold, coconut oil, cornmeal, cucumbers, blackberries, buttermilk, and clay among many others. Actually, you can mix a few of these ingredients and use it for a while to make your own new discoveries. I tell you the possibilities are endless.

There is really no better way for you to enjoy youthful skin that uses 100% natural homemade cleansers. It is actually helpful and very easy on your pockets.

Conclusion

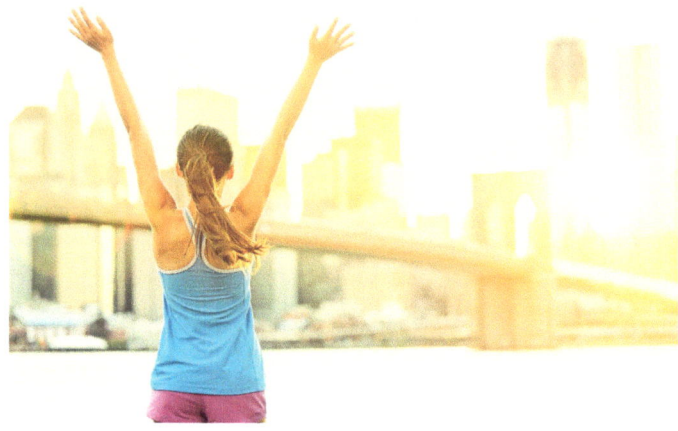

I hope you now understand how important it is for you to eat, exercise and cleanse your skin if you want it to remain young and healthy for longer. Without a doubt this is the only way you can ensure youthful skin and body longevity.

Take the teachings in this e-book and make them habits. There is nothing better than adopting a helpful habit.

Once you make this e-book a habit, you will never have to worry about aging skin again.

Go ahead, dare to look ten years younger!

www.ingramcontent.com/pod-product-compliance
Lightning Source LLC
Chambersburg PA
CBHW050839290526
45792CB00001B/457